Misophonia

A Beginner's 2-Week Guide to Managing Misophonia Naturally, with a Sample Worksheet

copyright © 2022 Patrick Marshwell

All rights reserved No part of this book may be reproduced, or stored in a retrieval system, or transmitted in any form or by any means, electronic, mechanical, photocopying, recording, or otherwise, without express written permission of the publisher.

Disclaimer

By reading this disclaimer, you are accepting the terms of the disclaimer in full. If you disagree with this disclaimer, please do not read the guide.

All of the content within this guide is provided for informational and educational purposes only, and should not be accepted as independent medical or other professional advice. The author is not a doctor, physician, nurse, mental health provider, or registered nutritionist/dietician. Therefore, using and reading this guide does not establish any form of a physician-patient relationship.

Always consult with a physician or another qualified health provider with any issues or questions you might have regarding any sort of medical condition. Do not ever disregard any qualified professional medical advice or delay seeking that advice because of anything you have read in this guide. The information in this guide is not intended to be any sort of medical advice and should not be used in lieu of any medical advice by a licensed and qualified medical professional.

The information in this guide has been compiled from a variety of known sources. However, the author cannot attest to or guarantee the accuracy of each source and thus should not be held liable for any errors or omissions.

You acknowledge that the publisher of this guide will not be held liable for any loss or damage of any kind incurred as a result of this guide or the reliance on any information provided within this guide. You acknowledge and agree that you assume all risk and responsibility for any action you undertake in response to the information in this guide.

Using this guide does not guarantee any particular result (e.g., weight loss or a cure). By reading this guide, you acknowledge that there are no guarantees to any specific outcome or results you can expect.

All product names, diet plans, or names used in this guide are for identification purposes only and are the property of their respective owners. The use of these names does not imply endorsement. All other trademarks cited herein are the property of their respective owners.

Where applicable, this guide is not intended to be a substitute for the original work of this diet plan and is, at most, a supplement to the original work for this diet plan and never a direct substitute. This guide is a personal expression of the facts of that diet plan.

Where applicable, persons shown in the cover images are stock photography models and the publisher has obtained the rights to use the images through license agreements with third-party stock image companies.

Table of Contents

Introduction	6
All About Misophonia	9
Trigger Sounds	10
Symptoms	11
Risk Factors and Causes	13
Diagnosis	15
Managing Misophonia	16
Wearing Earplugs or Noise-Canceling Headphones	16
Create a Misophonia-Free Zone in Your Home	18
Avoid possible trigger places	21
What if I can't avoid my trigger sounds?	21
Counseling and Therapy	23
How does cognitive behavioral therapy work?	24
Relaxation Techniques	25
Sound Sensitivity Training, a 2-Week Guide	34
Week 1 – Getting Started in Sound Sensitivity Training	36
Create a Trigger List	36
Rate the Trigger Sounds	39
Prepare a sound sensitivity rating guide	43
Doing the Exercise	45
Week 2 – Progressing in Sound Sensitivity Training	46
Remember to take a break	46
Stay motivated and focused	50
Return to your doctor for a follow-up consultation	55
Why Does Sound Sensitivity Training Work?	56
Talk to Friends and Family	61
Conclusion	63
Sample Worksheets	66
FAQs	68
References and Helpful Links	71

Introduction

Misophonia is a condition that significantly impacts the lives of those who suffer from it. They experience intense emotional reactions to specific sounds, often ones that are considered normal or even mundane by others.

For individuals with misophonia, everyday noises such as chewing, tapping, or even breathing can trigger feelings of anger, anxiety, or distress. This guide aims to provide a comprehensive overview of misophonia, offering insights into its causes, symptoms, and potential coping strategies.

The world is full of various sounds and noises, many of which blend into the background of daily life. However, for a person with misophonia, certain sounds stand out in a way that is both disruptive and distressing.

The sounds that trigger these reactions are typically repetitive and are linked with negative emotions. The impact of misophonia can extend to personal relationships, work environments, and overall quality of life. Understanding this condition is crucial for both those who suffer from it and those who interact with it.

What causes misophonia? Though the exact origins remain unclear, researchers suggest that it may be linked to the brain's limbic system, which is responsible for regulating emotions. When people with misophonia hear a trigger sound, their brains seem to overreact, leading to extreme emotional responses. These reactions can range from irritation and discomfort to outright rage and panic.

Misophonia often starts in childhood or adolescence and can persist into adulthood. It is not uncommon for individuals with misophonia to feel misunderstood or dismissed by others, making it essential to raise awareness about the condition. Increased understanding can help reduce the stigma and support those affected in finding effective coping mechanisms.

Living with misophonia can be challenging, but there are ways to manage and alleviate its impact. Cognitive-behavioral therapy (CBT) has shown promise in helping individuals reframe their reactions to trigger sounds. Techniques such as mindfulness and relaxation exercises can also be beneficial in reducing stress and improving emotional regulation.

For some, finding practical solutions can make a significant difference. Noise-canceling headphones, soundproofing living spaces, and creating quiet zones can help minimize exposure to trigger sounds. Additionally, educating friends, family, and colleagues about misophonia can foster a more supportive and empathetic environment.

As awareness grows, so does the availability of resources and support for those with misophonia. Online communities, support groups, and professional organizations offer valuable information and connections for individuals and their families. These platforms provide a space to share experiences, seek advice, and find solidarity among those who understand the unique challenges of misophonia.

In this beginner's quick start guide, you will discover…

- What misophonia is all about
- Its symptoms and what it feels like
- The possible trigger sounds and risk factors
- A 2-week plan on how to manage misophonia
- How it's diagnosed and treated
- How to manage misophonia

By exploring the causes, symptoms, and coping strategies outlined in this guide, readers will gain a deeper understanding of misophonia and how to navigate life with this condition. Whether you are personally affected or know someone who is, this comprehensive guide aims to equip you with the knowledge and tools needed to manage misophonia effectively.

All About Misophonia

Misophonia is a condition where certain sounds trigger negative emotions and feelings of anxiety. Mainly, it triggers a fight-or-flight response that can be debilitating, making it hard to function in day-to-day life. For example, the sound of someone chewing might make you feel angry or disgusted.

In a way, we all have a specific noise or sound we can't stand. It could be the sound made by scraping utensils on plates or pans, constantly knocking on a surface, or scratching nails on a chalkboard to name a few. However, for people who don't suffer from misophonia, despite the immediate negative response they feel from hearing these sounds, they are somewhat able to control their feelings and reactions. Their annoyance with the noise also decreases over time.

For those with misophonia, the negative sensations they feel happen regularly, even on sounds that other people barely hear. Perhaps due to this, as well as the fact that their reactions are usually intense and may seem an overreaction by others, they tend to just keep to themselves and not talk about their condition.

At the moment, experts don't know much about this condition because of several factors. Those who have them don't necessarily talk about them with their doctors, so the healthcare providers aren't usually familiar with them. Because it's not fairly known to most people, there may also be some stigma formed against those with misophonia. This may result in some patients feeling embarrassed about their condition, so they don't openly talk about the symptoms they're experiencing.

The scientific community still hasn't included misophonia in its list of disorders due to its novelty and the lack of scientific research and case studies regarding it. However, this doesn't mean the condition is left untreated by doctors. Usually, patients initially get help to understand their condition, as well as identify what exactly triggers them as well as how much they are affected by these sounds.

Trigger Sounds

Most people with misophonia have specific "trigger" sounds that bother them. These triggers can be different for each person, but some common ones include:

- chewing or eating noises
- gulping or swallowing noises
- breathing noises
- footsteps
- coughing

- clicking or tapping sounds

People with misophonia often feel the need to flee or fight when they hear these trigger sounds. This can lead to avoidance behaviors, such as:

- Leaving a room when someone is eating
- Wearing earplugs or headphones in public
- Asking people to stop making certain noises

Misophonia can also cause difficulty in personal relationships. For example, you might avoid social situations out of fear that you'll be triggered. Or, if you're triggered by a sound your partner makes, it can lead to arguments and resentment.

Symptoms

Describing the symptoms of misophonia can be somewhat complex. The primary symptom is an intensely negative reaction to specific triggering sounds. However, this condition is not limited to just that.

The responses to these triggering sounds can vary widely and are not confined to feelings of anger or frustration. Some common negative emotions experienced include:

- *Aggression*: An urge to take forceful action against the source of the sound.

- *Anger*: A strong feeling of displeasure or hostility triggered by the sound.
- *Annoyance*: Mild irritation that can escalate with repeated exposure to the triggering noise.
- *Disgust*: A profound sense of repulsion or aversion to the sound.
- *Irritation*: Persistent discomfort or agitation caused by exposure to the noise.
- *Nervousness*: A state of anxiety or unease provoked by the trigger sound.
- *Rage*: Intense anger that might lead to a loss of control.
- *Uneasiness*: A general feeling of discomfort or apprehension when hearing the sound.

In addition to these emotional responses, individuals with misophonia may also experience anxious or panicky feelings, as if they are trapped or losing control. The intensity of these reactions often depends on the significance of the trigger sounds to the person.

Beyond emotional symptoms, there are also physical sensations associated with misophonia, such as:

- *A desire to physically or verbally lash out when feeling aggressive*: This can manifest as a compulsion to shout or strike out in response to the triggering sound.

- ***Chest or body pain, typically a sensation of tightness or intense pressure***: Individuals might feel a constricting sensation in their chest or other parts of their body.
- ***Increases in blood pressure, heart rate, and body temperature***: These physiological responses indicate the body's heightened state of arousal and stress.

An article published on Nature.com by psychiatrists outlines the following points about misophonia within the field of psychiatry:

1. Pronounced mental suffering of patients
2. The cognitive (obsessive) and affective nature of the symptoms following conditioning
3. Behavioral coping strategies such as avoidance
4. Treatment options within the realm of psychiatric discipline

The goal of these psychiatrists is to support the study of detecting neurobiological mechanisms that may assist in recognizing and accepting misophonia as a legitimate disorder.

Risk Factors and Causes

The exact causes of misophonia remain unclear, but several risk factors may contribute to its development. These include:

- *Family History*: Misophonia often runs in families, suggesting a genetic component. It may be passed down from generation to generation.
- *Anxiety or Depression*: Individuals with anxiety or depression seem to be more susceptible to developing misophonia. The heightened emotional sensitivity associated with these conditions might play a role.
- *Obsessive-Compulsive Disorder (OCD)*: Misophonia and OCD share some similar features, such as avoidance behaviors and obsessive thoughts. This overlap indicates that those with OCD may be at a higher risk.
- *Autism Spectrum Disorder*: Some research suggests that misophonia is more common among individuals with autism spectrum disorder. The heightened sensory sensitivities often associated with autism might contribute to the prevalence of misophonia in this group.
- *Gender*: There is some evidence indicating that misophonia is more common in women than in men.

Understanding these risk factors can help in identifying individuals who might be more likely to develop misophonia, thereby facilitating early intervention and management strategies.

Diagnosis

There are no formal criteria for diagnosing misophonia. However, your doctor may ask about your symptoms and how they're impacting your life. They may also do a physical exam to rule out other conditions with similar symptoms.

In the next chapters, we will cover some of the key strategies that can help you manage your misophonia naturally.

Managing Misophonia

Misophonia, even for experts, is still considered a novel condition. This is why, unfortunately, there is still no cure for it. However, there are treatments that can help you manage your symptoms and make day-to-day life more bearable.

If you have misophonia, there are a few things you can do to manage your condition and reduce your symptoms. One of the key ways to go about this is to avoid trigger sounds as much as you can. If possible, create a space where you can feel safe and get rid of the trigger sounds as best as possible.

Wearing Earplugs or Noise-Canceling Headphones

Start with the simplest solution: controlling what you can. This may involve wearing earplugs or noise-canceling headphones when you're exposed to bothersome sounds.

There is a variety of earplugs and noise-canceling headphones on the market, catering to different preferences and needs.

1. **Earplugs**

   Some people prefer foam earplugs, while others might find them uncomfortable. Here are examples of effective earplugs:

   - *Etymotic Research ER20XS*: Known for their high-fidelity sound reduction, these are great for those who need to filter out noise without compromising sound quality.
   - *Moldable Silicone Earplugs (e.g., Mack's Ear Plugs)*: These can be molded to fit the shape of your ear, providing a custom fit that blocks out noise effectively.
   - *Foam Earplugs (e.g., 3M E-A-Rsoft OCS1116)*: Commonly used and widely available, these foam earplugs expand to fill the ear canal and offer good noise reduction.

2. **Noise-Canceling Headphones**

   There are different styles of noise-canceling headphones, including over-the-ear and in-ear models. The primary difference between the two is that over-the-ear headphones cover the entire ear, while in-ear headphones fit into the ear canal.

   - *Over-the-Ear Headphones*: These tend to be more comfortable and effective at noise cancellation. However, they can be bulky and less portable. Examples include:

- ***Bose QuietComfort 25 Acoustic Noise Cancelling Headphones***: Renowned for their superior noise cancellation and comfort.
- ***Sennheiser PXC 550 Wireless Noise Cancelling Headphones***: These offer excellent sound quality and effective noise cancellation, along with the convenience of wireless connectivity.
- ***In-Ear Headphones***: More portable and generally less expensive, though they might not cancel noise as effectively as over-the-ear models. They can be a good option for those who need something lightweight and easy to carry.

If you're unsure which type of product to choose, consider reading online reviews or asking for recommendations from friends or family members. Trying out different options can help you find what works best for your specific needs and comfort levels.

Create a Misophonia-Free Zone in Your Home

Creating a misophonia-free zone in your home can significantly improve your quality of life by providing a sanctuary from triggering sounds. Here are some detailed steps to help you establish this space:

1. ***Identify a Quiet Area***: Start by selecting a part of your home that is naturally quieter and less frequented by other household members. This could be a spare bedroom, a study, or even a basement or attic space. The key is to choose an area where you can control the environment as much as possible.
2. ***Soundproofing***: Enhance the quietness of your chosen space by implementing soundproofing measures. Use heavy curtains or drapes on windows to block outside noise. Adding rugs or carpets can help absorb sound within the room. For more effective soundproofing, consider installing acoustic panels on the walls.
3. ***Communicate with Household Members***: Explain to your family and friends why it's important to maintain a quiet environment in this designated zone. Politely request that they avoid making specific noises (e.g., chewing, tapping, or loud conversations) when they are near or around this area. Clear communication about your needs can foster understanding and cooperation.
4. ***Set Up Your Space***: Arrange the room to create a comfortable and calming environment. Include any items that help you relax, such as comfortable seating, soft lighting, and perhaps even plants or artwork that you find soothing. Make this space your retreat where you can go to decompress and escape from triggering sounds.

5. ***Equip with Noise-Canceling Tools***: Always have noise-canceling headphones or earplugs readily available in your misophonia-free zone. These tools can provide additional layers of sound protection when needed. Invest in high-quality products that offer effective noise reduction and are comfortable for extended use.
6. ***Establish Boundaries***: Clearly define and enforce boundaries around your misophonia-free zone. Let household members know that when you are in this space, it is your time to unwind and escape from noise stressors. Consider setting up signals, like a closed door or a "do not disturb" sign, to indicate when you need uninterrupted quiet time.
7. ***Create a Routine***: Incorporate regular time in your misophonia-free zone into your daily routine. Whether it's for reading, meditating, working, or simply relaxing, consistent use of this space can help reduce overall stress and manage misophonia symptoms more effectively.
8. ***Maintenance and Adjustments***: Periodically assess your misophonia-free zone to ensure it continues to meet your needs. If certain noises start to intrude or if the space no longer feels as calming, make necessary adjustments. This might mean adding new soundproofing materials, rearranging the furniture, or updating your noise-canceling tools.

By taking these steps, you can create a haven in your home that offers relief from the distressing effects of misophonia. This dedicated space can serve as a crucial coping mechanism, allowing you to regain control over your auditory environment and improve your overall well-being.

Avoid possible trigger places

If possible, try to avoid places where you know there will be triggers, like restaurants or movie theaters. Other places you might want to avoid are ones where you can't control the noise level, such as offices or public transportation.

It's also important to understand that you can't always avoid trigger sounds. When this happens, there are a few things you can do to cope. Try to relax. Misophonia can cause a fight-or-flight response in your body, which makes it harder to think clearly. So, take a few deep breaths and try to focus on something else until the trigger sound goes away.

What if I can't avoid my trigger sounds?

If you can't avoid your trigger sounds, you can try to desensitize yourself to them. This is done by gradually exposing yourself to the sound in small increments until you're no longer bothered by it.

Desensitization is a form of exposure therapy, which is a type of treatment that's commonly used for anxiety disorders.

If you're interested in trying desensitization, there are a few things you can do:

1. Start by finding a recording of the sound that bothers you. You can usually find these online.
2. Once you have the recording, put it on at a very low volume. If it's too loud, you'll just end up feeling more anxious.
3. Listen to the sound for a few minutes and then take a break. Over time, you can gradually increase the volume until it's at a normal level.

It's important to note that desensitization can take time and patience. It might not work for everyone. It also may take a lot more than some sort of training. While you can give this a shot on your own, it's still best to consult with an expert or a therapist, so you can go about it in the best way possible.

Take note also that avoiding trigger sounds is not always possible. That's why it's important to have coping mechanisms in place to help you deal with the anxiety and stress that misophonia can cause. We'll cover some of these in the next chapter.

Counseling and Therapy

Talking to a counselor or therapist can help you learn how to deal with your reactions to trigger sounds. Some people find relief with cognitive behavioral therapy, which is a type of counseling that helps you change the way you think about and react to certain situations.

Cognitive-behavioral therapy is a type of counseling that helps you change the way you think about and react to certain situations. It is a short-term, goal-oriented form of therapy that is typically used to treat anxiety and depression.

If you have misophonia, you might find relief with cognitive behavioral therapy. This type of therapy can help you learn how to deal with your reactions to trigger sounds.

Cognitive-behavioral therapy is a talking therapy that can help you:

- understand your thoughts and feelings
- learn new ways of thinking and reacting
- manage stress
- cope with anxiety or depression

How does cognitive behavioral therapy work?

Cognitive-behavioral therapy usually involves meeting with a therapist for weekly sessions. You will discuss your thoughts, feelings, and behaviors during each session. The therapist will help you identify negative thought patterns and provide strategies for changing them.

For example, if you're afraid of trigger sounds, the therapist might help you challenge your beliefs about the sound. They might also teach you relaxation techniques to help you deal with your anxiety.

Cognitive-behavioral therapy is a short-term form of therapy that typically lasts for 10-12 weeks. It is considered to be one of the most effective treatments for anxiety and depression.

One of the reasons why CBT is so effective is that it addresses both the thoughts and the behaviors that are causing distress. For example, if someone is anxious about flying, CBT would help them to identify and challenge their negative thoughts about flying (e.g., "I'm going to crash"), as well as teach them coping strategies for dealing with their anxiety (e.g., deep breathing exercises).

CBT is also considered to be a very practical form of therapy. It is often conducted in a group setting, which can make it more affordable than individual therapy. Additionally, CBT can be done through self-help books and online programs, which makes it more accessible to people who may not be able to see a therapist regularly.

If you think cognitive behavioral therapy might be right for you, talk to your doctor or mental health professional about it.

If you are interested in finding a cognitive behavioral therapist, you can search for one in your area on the American Psychological Association website. Some other sources might include your insurance company or your local mental health center.

Relaxation Techniques

In addition to addressing negative thoughts and behaviors, cognitive-behavioral therapy also incorporates relaxation techniques to help manage anxiety. These can include;

Diaphragmatic breathing

There are a variety of relaxation techniques that can help you manage your misophonia. Some people find relief with diaphragmatic breathing, which is a type of deep breathing that helps you relax.

Diaphragmatic breathing is a type of deep breathing that is often used as a relaxation technique. It involves breathing deeply from the diaphragm, which is the muscle located at the base of your lungs. This muscle is responsible for pumping air in and out of your lungs. The diaphragm is made up of two layers of muscle—the upper and lower layers. The upper layer of the diaphragm is called the dome, while the lower layer is called the coastal arch.

The diaphragm is attached to your ribs at the costal arch. When you breathe in, the diaphragm contracts and moves downward. This action creates a vacuum within your chest cavity, which causes air to be drawn into your lungs. When you breathe out, the diaphragm relaxes and moves upward. This action forces air out of your lungs.

The main function of the diaphragm is to help you breathe. However, the diaphragm also plays a role in other body functions, such as digestion and urination.

The diaphragm is an important muscle in your body and it is essential for proper breathing. This type of breathing can help to oxygenate your blood and relax your body.

There are a few different ways that you can practice diaphragmatic breathing. One way is to sit in a comfortable position with your back straight and place one hand on your stomach. Breathe in slowly through your nose, allowing your stomach to expand. As you exhale, tighten your abdominal muscles and push all of the air out through your mouth.

Another way to practice diaphragmatic breathing is to lie down on your back with one hand on your stomach and the other on your chest. Breathe in slowly through your nose, allowing your stomach to rise. As you exhale, push all of the air out through your mouth and feel your stomach fall.

You can also practice diaphragmatic breathing while walking. Simply focus on taking deep breaths from your diaphragm as you walk.

If you're having trouble breathing from your diaphragm, place a small book or another small object on your stomach and focus on pushing it up as you inhale.

Once you've mastered the basic technique of diaphragmatic breathing, you can start to experiment with different ways to use it. For example, you can try breathing deeply for a count of four and then exhaling for a count of eight. Or, you can breathe in for a count of four and then hold your breath for a count of seven before exhaling.

There are many different ways that you can use diaphragmatic breathing to help reduce stress and anxiety. Experiment with different techniques and find the ones that work best.

Why does diaphragmatic breathing work?

When you breathe deeply from your diaphragm, it massages your vagus nerve. This is the longest cranial nerve in your body and it extends from your brainstem to your abdomen. The vagus nerve is responsible for controlling many of the involuntary functions of your body, such as heart rate and digestion.

The cranial nerve is also connected to your limbic system, which is the part of your brain that controls emotions. This is why deep breathing from your diaphragm can help to decrease stress and anxiety. In addition to massaging your vagus nerve, deep breathing also increases the amount of oxygen in your blood. This can help to improve brain function and increase overall energy levels.

There are a few reasons why having more oxygen in your blood is important. First, oxygen is essential for the proper function of all cells in the body. Without enough oxygen, cells will begin to die and organs will start to fail.

Additionally, oxygen is necessary for the body to produce energy. When there is not enough oxygen in the blood, the body will not be able to produce energy efficiently and will become fatigued more easily. Finally, oxygen plays a role in detoxifying the blood. When there is not enough oxygen present, toxins, and waste products can build up in the blood, leading to potentially dangerous health problems.

Finally, diaphragmatic breathing helps to activate your parasympathetic nervous system. This is the part of your nervous system responsible for rest and digestion. When you're stressed, your sympathetic nervous system is activated, which can lead to an increase in heart rate and blood pressure. Activating your parasympathetic nervous system can help to counteract the effects

Massaging the vagus nerve with deep breathing can help to decrease stress and anxiety. It can also help to improve mood, increase energy levels, and promote relaxation. Diaphragmatic breathing is a simple and effective way to reduce stress and anxiety.

Muscle Relaxation

Another relaxation technique is progressive muscle relaxation. This is a technique that involves tensing and relaxing different muscle groups in your body.

To practice progressive muscle relaxation, start by tensing the muscles in your feet for a count of five. Then, relax the muscles for a count of five. Continue this process moving up through your body, working your way from your feet to your head.

As you tense each muscle group, focus on the sensation of the muscle contracting. As you relax the muscle group, focus on the sensation of the muscle release.

It's important to tense and relax each muscle group slowly and smoothly. Don't hold your breath as you tense or relax the muscles.

Besides the feet, you can also tense and relax the following muscle groups:

- calves
- thighs

- hips
- arms
- shoulders
- neck
- face

Progressive muscle relaxation is a simple and effective way to reduce stress and anxiety. It can also help to improve sleep quality and reduce pain.

Progressive muscle relaxation can help to reduce stress and anxiety. It can also help to improve sleep quality and promote overall relaxation.

There are many different relaxation techniques that you can use to reduce stress and anxiety. Experiment with different techniques and find the ones that work best for you.

Meditation

Meditation is another relaxation technique that can be helpful in managing stress and anxiety. Meditation involves focusing on your breath and letting thoughts pass through your mind without judgment.

If you're interested in meditation, there are many ways to get started. You can find a local class, download an app, or follow a video. Or, you can simply sit down and start meditating on your own.

Here are a few tips to help you get started:

1. ***Find a comfortable place to sit or lie down.*** You don't need to be in a special position to meditate, but it should be comfortable so that you can remain still for a while.
2. ***Close your eyes and focus on your breath.*** Once you're settled, close your eyes and focus on your breathing. Simply observe the rise and fall of your chest as you inhale and exhale.
3. ***Let go of your thoughts.*** As you focus on your breath, you may find that your mind starts to wander. When this happens, simply try to let go of the thoughts and return your focus to your breathing.
4. ***Be patient.*** Meditation takes practice, so don't be discouraged if it's not easy at first. Just keep at it and eventually, you'll find that it gets easier and more enjoyable.
5. ***Make it a daily habit.*** The best way to benefit from meditation is to do it every day. Even just a few minutes of meditation can make a difference. Just repeat the meditation process that you found helpful or effective daily.

If you find it difficult to focus on your breath, you can try counting each time you inhale and exhale. You can also try focusing on a mantra or affirmation.

Guided Imagery

Guided imagery is a relaxation technique that leverages the power of your imagination to create a serene environment, providing a mental escape from the stresses of daily life.

To practice, begin by finding a quiet, comfortable place where you won't be disturbed. Sit or lie down, close your eyes, and take a few deep, calming breaths. Feel the tension leaving your body with each exhale.

Next, visualize yourself in a peaceful setting—perhaps a sunlit beach with waves gently lapping at the shore, a tranquil forest with the sound of birds chirping and leaves rustling in the breeze, or even your backyard, filled with the familiar scents and sounds that bring you comfort and joy.

As you concentrate on this image, immerse yourself in the details. What do you see? Is the sky a brilliant blue, or is it adorned with fluffy white clouds? What do you hear? The rhythmic sound of the ocean, the whispering of the wind through the trees, or the melody of birdsong? What do you smell? The salty tang of the sea air, the earthy scent of pine needles, or the fragrant aroma of blooming flowers?

Allow yourself to fully experience this peaceful place. If your mind starts to wander, gently redirect your focus back to the image, reassuring yourself that it's okay to take this time for relaxation and mental rejuvenation.

Guided imagery can effectively reduce stress and anxiety, enhance sleep quality, and promote overall relaxation. By regularly practicing this technique, you may find that it becomes easier to tap into this serene state of mind, helping you to better manage the pressures of everyday life and improve your overall well-being.

Sound Sensitivity Training, a 2-Week Guide

Even at home or on your own, you can try doing exercises to help you manage misophonia. Now that you've learned some relaxation techniques, you can include this in your training or exercise to manage misophonia, in the comforts of your home.

During the first week, you can start exploring ways to create an effective method for managing your condition. Before you begin, make sure that you have at least tried the relaxation techniques listed in the previous chapter. It's also highly advised that you discuss this with your doctor or therapist so that they can help you create a plan or strategy for managing misophonia at home.

Before we proceed with the first week of this exercise, here's information about sound sensitivity training.

In addition to that, there's another approach that can help manage misophonia, which is called sound sensitivity training. This is a process of gradually exposing yourself to the sounds that trigger your misophonia. This is different from desensitization, which involves exposure to the trigger sound at a loud level.

Sound sensitivity training should be done gradually and at a level that is tolerable for you. The goal is to help you become more tolerant of the trigger sounds and to reduce your reactivity to them.

Week 1 – Getting Started in Sound Sensitivity Training

For starters, this training will not completely guarantee to treat the condition. However, as you go along the training, getting used to being exposed to the trigger sounds may eventually help you deal with it regularly.

Create a Trigger List

One of the first steps in sound sensitivity training is creating a comprehensive trigger list. This initial task is crucial for identifying the specific sounds that trigger your misophonia and will form the foundation for your training exercises. Here's how to get started:

1. **Spend Time Observing**
   - ***Daily Activities***: Pay close attention to your daily activities and interactions to identify sounds that consistently cause discomfort or irritation. These could occur at home, work, or in social settings.
   - ***Note Situations***: Be mindful of situations where you feel particularly stressed or annoyed by certain sounds.

For instance, during meals, in meetings, or while commuting.

2. **Document Your Findings**
- *Notebook/Piece of Paper*: Write down each triggering sound in a dedicated notebook or on a piece of paper. Keeping a physical record allows for easy reference and tracking over time.
- *Digital Options*: If you prefer, you can also use digital tools like note apps on your phone or computer to keep track of your triggers. The key is to have a detailed list that you can update and review regularly.

3. **Be Specific**
- *Detail Each Sound*: Be as specific as possible when listing your triggers. Instead of just writing "chewing," note whether it's crunchy foods, gum chewing, or slurping that bothers you.
- *Environmental Context*: Consider the context in which these sounds occur. Are they more bothersome when you're in a quiet room versus a noisy environment?

4. **Identify the Examples of Common Triggers**
- *Chewing*: Distinguish between different types of chewing sounds, such as loud or soft chewing, and note if it's more disturbing when made by specific individuals.
- *Tapping*: Identify different tapping sounds, like fingers tapping on a table, pen clicking, or foot tapping.

- *Breathing*: Note whether heavy breathing, snoring, or nose whistling triggers your misophonia.
- *Other Sounds*: Include less common triggers like typing on a keyboard, rustling paper, or specific animal noises.

5. **Categorize and Rate**
- *Organize Sounds*: Once you have a list of triggers, you might find it helpful to categorize them based on their intensity or the setting in which they occur.
- *Initial Ratings*: Though formally rating the sounds comes later, you can start with an informal assessment to prioritize which sounds to tackle first.

6. **Regular Updates**
- *Ongoing Process*: Recognize that identifying triggers is an ongoing process. New triggers may emerge over time, so make it a habit to update your list regularly.
- *Review Often*: Periodically review your trigger list to ensure it remains accurate and comprehensive as you progress through your sound sensitivity training.

By dedicating time to meticulously creating and maintaining a trigger list, you lay a solid foundation for your sound sensitivity training. This methodical approach not only helps in identifying the specific sounds that trigger your misophonia but also provides a structured way to monitor and manage your progress effectively.

Rate the Trigger Sounds

Once you have a comprehensive list of the trigger sounds that bother you, the next crucial step is to rate each sound based on how triggering it is for you. This rating will help you systematically approach your sound sensitivity training.

Rating the Trigger Sounds

1. *Use a 1-10 Scale*
   - <u>Definition</u>: Rate each sound on a scale from 1 to 10, where 1 represents the least triggering and 10 represents the most triggering.
   - <u>Consistency</u>: Ensure you apply this scale consistently across all your identified triggers. This will provide a clear picture of which sounds are more challenging for you.

2. *Consider Emotional and Physical Reactions*
   - <u>Emotional Impact</u>: Reflect on how each sound makes you feel emotionally. Does it cause mild annoyance, significant discomfort, or extreme irritation?
   - <u>Physical Responses</u>: Note any physical reactions you experience, such as increased heart rate, muscle tension, or even headaches. These responses can help you accurately rate the intensity of each trigger.

3. *Examples of Ratings*

- *Chewing*: Chewing might be rated as a 3 if it causes moderate discomfort but is generally manageable.
- *Tapping*: Tapping could be rated as a 2 if it is mildly irritating but not overwhelming.
- *Breathing*: Heavy breathing might be rated as a 4 if it consistently disrupts your focus and causes significant stress.

4. *Focus on Lower-Level Triggers*
   - *Initial Focus*: For the first week, concentrate on the sounds rated at a level 4 or below. These lower-level triggers will be easier to start with and will help you build resilience gradually.
   - *Gradual Progression*: Starting with less intense sounds allows you to acclimate to the exposure therapy without feeling overwhelmed. As you become more comfortable, you can gradually move on to higher-rated sounds in subsequent weeks.

Preparing the Recordings

1. *Find or Create Recordings*
   - *Online Resources*: Many common trigger sounds can be found online through websites, apps, or platforms like YouTube. Search for high-quality recordings that accurately represent the triggering sounds.

- *Personal Recordings*: If specific sounds are not available online, consider recording them yourself using a smartphone or other recording device. Ensure the recordings are clear and free from background noise to maximize their effectiveness.

2. **Multiple Sources**
   - *Variety*: Collect multiple recordings of the same sound from different sources to ensure variety. This can prevent habituation and help you better generalize your tolerance to similar sounds in different contexts.

3. **Organize Your Recordings**
   - *Categorization*: Organize your recordings by trigger type and intensity level. This will make it easier to access and use them during your exercises.
   - *Labeling*: Clearly label each recording with the trigger sound and its rating to avoid confusion during your training sessions.

Implement Frequency Exercise

1. **Structured Sessions**
   - *30-Second Exercises*: Start with brief exposure sessions. Play the recordings for 30 seconds, followed by a 30-second break. This approach

helps you get accustomed to the sounds without overwhelming yourself.
- *Adjust Duration*: If 30 seconds feels too long initially, reduce the duration to a level that is more comfortable for you and gradually increase it over time.

2. **Example Schedule**
   - *Morning Session*: Listen to each chosen sound for 30 seconds, take a 30-second break, and repeat. Conduct this exercise twice daily.
   - *Evening Session*: Repeat the same exercise in the evening for consistency and reinforcement.

Take Notes

1. **Document Experiences**
   - *Immediate Reactions*: After each session, write down your immediate emotional and physical reactions to the trigger sounds.
   - *Progress Over Time*: Track any changes in your tolerance levels throughout the week. Note improvements, challenges, and any adjustments made to your training plan.

2. **Detailed Observations**
   - *Emotional Response*: Describe how the sound made you feel (e.g., anxious, irritated, neutral).

- *Physical Response*: Note any physical reactions (e.g., increased heart rate, tension).
- *Effectiveness of Training*: Assess how effective the exposure sessions were in reducing your sensitivity to the sounds.

By systematically rating your trigger sounds and preparing targeted exposure exercises, you can create a structured and effective plan for managing misophonia. This methodical approach not only helps in tracking progress but also provides a clear way to make necessary adjustments for better outcomes.

Prepare a sound sensitivity rating guide

Use this sample template to help you with this exercise. In making a sound sensitivity template, make sure that you are able to keep track and make notes on each trigger sound, especially during your sound sensitivity therapy. This way, you can modify or tweak the process according to your preferences and experiences.

Trigger Sound List	Sensitivity Rate	Frequency Exercise	Notes

The sample sound sensitivity template below takes notes of the following:

1. *Trigger sound list*: List down the sounds that trigger your misophonia
2. *Sensitivity rate*: Rate each trigger sound, with 10 being the most triggering. If possible, try to list down your trigger sounds from the least triggering to the worst. That way, you can slowly work down your list in an organized manner.
3. *Frequency exercise*: This column is most likely the modifiable one. You can either take note of the time/s of the day when you're supposed to work on the particular trigger sound, or you can also tally the number of times you worked on the particular sound during your therapy. Just make sure that you impose a consistent training-break rule. What's suggested above is a 30-second exercise and a 30-second break. However, in the beginning, you can do it for a shorter time if half a minute is too long for you.
4. *Notes*: Write down your experiences, challenges, and other important information that you think would be beneficial while you're doing your therapy or exercise. Make sure that you go over your notes regularly, so you can modify or adapt your method to make it more effective, especially as you progress to the higher-rated sounds.

Doing the Exercise

Once you have found a recording of the sound, put on some headphones and start at a low volume. Listen to the sound for 30 seconds and then take a break for 30 seconds. Try to figure out just how frequently you can deal with doing the exercise for each sound.

As you listen to the sound, pay attention to your reactions and emotions. What do you feel? What do you think? Are you able to tolerate the sound? Make notes on these observations, and try also to gauge just how much you can handle per day.

If you've considered doing this exercise for a specific number of hours daily or on certain days of the week, check also just how many trigger sounds you think you can handle per exercise. Write that down on your notes and make sure you stick to that.

Because it's only your first week, expect some drawbacks and a rough start. The sounds will definitely trigger you but don't get discouraged. Pace yourself slowly so you can eventually progress. Remember that exercises like this one are not one-size-fits-all. Your progress will be different from everyone else's.

Week 2 – Progressing in Sound Sensitivity Training

During the second week, it can be expected that somehow, you've either progressed on your trigger sound list—working on the trigger sounds that ranked higher on your triggers—or you have somehow gotten a bit used to hearing some of your trigger sounds without experiencing intensely negative reactions.

Just as mentioned previously, progress on this training or exercise will not be the same for everyone, so don't pressure yourself too much. As long as you're consistently working on your trigger sound list, you are making progress.

Remember to take a break

Sound sensitivity training can be challenging, and it's essential to approach it with a balanced mindset. Taking breaks and gradually increasing exposure are critical components for successful progress. Here's a detailed guide on how to manage your sessions effectively:

Tolerance and Breaks

1. *Monitor Your Tolerance*
   - *Tune into Your Reactions*: Pay close attention to your emotional and physical responses during each exposure session. If you find the sound overwhelming or intolerable, it's important to acknowledge this without pushing yourself too hard.
   - *Gradual Exposure*: Building tolerance takes time. Start with shorter durations and lower volumes if necessary, and increase them gradually as you become more comfortable.

2. *Take a Break*
   - *Step Away*: If a particular sound becomes too much to handle, take a break. Step away from the exercise and engage in a calming activity to reset your stress levels.
   - *Duration of Breaks*: The length of the break can vary based on your needs. It could be a few minutes to an hour or longer, depending on how much time you need to feel ready to try again.

3. *Try Again Later*
   - *Resume When Ready*: Once you feel more at ease, try the exposure exercise again. The key is to maintain consistency while respecting your limits.

- *Adjustments*: If you continue to find the sound intolerable, consider shortening the exposure duration or lowering the volume further until you build more resilience.

Gradually Increase Volume

1. *Start Low*
   - *Initial Volume*: Begin with the volume set to a level that is barely noticeable but still audible. This helps ease you into the exposure without causing immediate discomfort.
   - *Baseline Comfort*: Establish a baseline volume that you find minimally triggering and use this as your starting point.

2. *Incremental Increases*
   - *Small Steps*: Gradually increase the volume in small increments over several sessions. This slow progression allows your nervous system to adapt without feeling overwhelmed.
   - *Monitor Reactions*: Keep track of your reactions at each new volume level. If a particular increase is too much, scale back slightly and try again at a later time.

Incorporate Relaxation Techniques

3. *Use Learned Techniques*

- *Previous Chapter Methods*: Apply relaxation techniques you learned in the previous chapter to help manage stress and anxiety during breaks and exercises. These might include deep breathing, progressive muscle relaxation, or guided imagery.
- *Immediate Relief*: Utilize these techniques immediately after a sound exposure session to calm your mind and body before taking a break.

4. **Integration During Breaks**
   - *Calming Activities*: Engage in activities that help you relax during your breaks, such as listening to soothing music, practicing mindfulness, or doing gentle yoga stretches.
   - *Prepare for Re-Exposure*: Use relaxation methods just before resuming an exposure session to enter the exercise in a calm and centered state.

Progressing to Higher-Rated Sounds

1. ***Build Confidence***
   - *Celebrate Successes*: Acknowledge and celebrate your progress with lower-rated sounds. Each step forward builds confidence and prepares you for more challenging triggers.

- *Reinforce Tolerance*: Periodically revisit previously mastered sounds to reinforce your tolerance and ensure lasting progress.

2. **Gradual Transition**
    - *Incremental Steps*: As you become more tolerant of lower-rated sounds, begin to introduce sounds with slightly higher ratings. Follow the same gradual exposure and break-taking process.
    - *Regular Reviews*: Regularly review your notes and experiences to adjust your approach as needed. If a higher-rated sound becomes too challenging, it's okay to step back and spend more time on lower-rated sounds before trying again.

By taking breaks when needed, gradually increasing volume, and integrating relaxation techniques, you create a sustainable and adaptive approach to sound sensitivity training. This method not only helps in managing your misophonia but also supports your overall well-being throughout the process.

Stay motivated and focused

Sound sensitivity training is a journey that requires patience, persistence, and self-compassion. Staying motivated and focused can make a significant difference in your progress.

Here's how to maintain a positive and balanced approach throughout your training:

Gradual Progression
1. *Take It One Step at a Time*
    - *Small Steps*: Understand that progress should be gradual. Start with less triggering sounds and slowly work your way up to more challenging ones.
    - *Short Sessions*: Begin with shorter exposure sessions, such as 10-15 seconds, if 30 seconds feels too long. Increase the duration incrementally as you build tolerance.

2. *Set Realistic Goals*
    - *Achievable Milestones*: Set small, realistic goals for each week. For example, aim to increase the duration of exposure by 5 seconds after a few successful sessions.
    - *Celebrate Successes*: Celebrate each milestone you achieve, no matter how small. Recognizing your progress helps build confidence and motivation.

Self-Pacing
1. *Listen to Your Body*
    - *Monitor Stress Levels*: Pay attention to your physical and emotional responses during

exercises. If you start to feel overwhelmed, it's a signal to take a break.
- *Adjust as Needed*: Modify the intensity, duration, or frequency of your exercises based on your comfort level. There's no rush; what matters is a steady, sustainable improvement.

2. **Don't Push Too Hard**
   - *Avoid Overexertion*: Pushing yourself too hard can lead to increased stress and anxiety, which can be counterproductive. It's better to make slow, steady progress than to risk burnout.
   - *Balance Effort with Rest*: Ensure you balance your practice sessions with adequate relaxation to prevent feeling overwhelmed.

Motivation and Focus

1. ***Keep a Journal***
   - *Track Progress*: Maintain a journal to record your experiences, challenges, and achievements. Regularly reviewing your entries can illuminate how far you've come and keep you motivated.
   - *Reflect on Positives*: Focus on the positive changes you notice, even if they seem minor. Small improvements add up over time.

2. ***Stay Positive***

- *Positive Reinforcement*: Use positive reinforcement by rewarding yourself for reaching milestones. Rewards can be anything that makes you happy, like a favorite treat or a relaxing activity.
- *Affirmations*: Use positive affirmations to boost your confidence. Remind yourself that you're capable and making progress.

3. Professional Support

- *Therapists*: Consider seeking support from a therapist who specializes in misophonia or sound sensitivity. Professional guidance can provide personalized strategies and encouragement.
- *Support Groups*: Join support groups or online communities where you can share experiences and advice with others who understand your challenges.

4. Mindfulness Practices

- *Mindfulness Exercises*: Incorporate mindfulness practices into your routine to help manage stress and stay focused. Techniques like meditation, deep breathing, and progressive muscle relaxation can be beneficial.
- *Stay Present*: Practice staying present during exposure exercises. Focusing on the current

moment can reduce anxiety about future discomfort.

Flexibility and Patience
1. *Be Flexible*
   - *Adapt Strategies*: Be open to adjusting your strategies based on what works best for you. Everyone's journey is unique, and what works for one person might need tweaking for another.
   - *Experiment*: Don't be afraid to experiment with different approaches to find what helps you the most.

2. *Practice Self-Compassion*
   - *Kindness to Self*: Treat yourself with kindness and understanding. Misophonia can be challenging, but being hard on yourself will only add to the stress.
   - *Accept Setbacks*: Accept that there may be setbacks along the way. Progress is not always linear, and that's okay. What matters is your overall trend toward improvement.

By maintaining a gradual, self-paced approach, staying motivated, and focusing on positive changes, you can effectively manage your sound sensitivity training. Remember, this is a marathon, not a sprint. Being kind to yourself and celebrating your progress will help you stay on track and achieve your goals.

Return to your doctor for a follow-up consultation

Once you're done with the 2-week program, schedule a visit to your doctor or therapist, and let them know how the training exercise helped you. Share with them your notes or the rating guide you used. This way, your doctor may have an idea of how effective sound sensitivity therapy is, and how you may go about this later.

If you find that sound sensitivity training is causing you more stress, take a break and try another approach. It's always great to go back to your doctor and seek assistance. Show them your notes during your sound sensitivity training as these may help them assess you better and provide you with better options, either in doing the same exercise or trying out a different one.

This type of therapy can help you get used to the sound of your triggers so they don't bother you as much. With sound sensitivity training, you'll slowly and gradually expose yourself to your trigger sounds for a short period of time each day. Over time, you should find that the sound doesn't bother you as much.

Why Does Sound Sensitivity Training Work?

Sound sensitivity training, also known as exposure therapy, operates on several key principles that can help reduce overall noise anxiety and increase comfort in loud environments. Here's a detailed look at why this approach is effective:

Desensitization of the Nervous System

1. *Repeated Exposure*
    - *Consistency*: The core concept of sound sensitivity training is the repeated, controlled exposure to slightly louder sounds over time. This repeated exposure helps desensitize the ears and the nervous system to the sensation of sound.
    - *Gradual Acclimation*: Just as people with a fear of heights may gradually feel more relaxed after repeatedly standing on tall buildings or bridges, individuals with sound sensitivity can become more tolerant of specific noises through consistent exposure.

2. *Neurological Adaptation*
    - *Habituation*: Over time, the brain and nervous system begin to habituate to the sounds. This means that the sounds become less novel and alarming, reducing the intensity of the emotional and physical reactions they provoke.

- *Threshold Adjustment*: The threshold for what constitutes a "triggering" sound can shift, making everyday noises less distressing.

Gradual Increase in Volume

1. **Controlled Environment**
   - *Safe Settings*: By gradually increasing the volume of sounds in a controlled environment, the brain is given the opportunity to adapt without feeling overwhelmed. This process is carefully managed to ensure it remains within the individual's tolerance levels.
   - *Incremental Steps*: Incremental increases in volume allow for a step-by-step approach, preventing sudden jumps that could cause setbacks.

2. **Lessening the Startle Response**
   - *Predictable Patterns*: When sounds are introduced gradually and predictably, the brain learns to anticipate them, which can significantly lessen the startle response. This anticipation reduces the shock value of unexpected loud noises.
   - *Enhanced Control*: Feeling in control of the exposure process can also diminish anxiety. Knowing that you can stop or lower the sound if

it becomes too much helps build confidence and reduces fear.

Change in Perception and Attitude

1. *Cognitive Shifts*
   - <u>Reframing Noise</u>: As individuals become more comfortable with slightly loud sounds, their overall attitude and perception of noise can shift. They may start to see these sounds as manageable rather than threatening.
   - <u>Positive Associations</u>: Positive experiences with controlled exposure can replace negative associations with certain sounds, leading to a more relaxed attitude towards them.

2. *Reduced Negative Impact*
   - <u>Improved Tolerance</u>: Increased tolerance to sounds means that noise has less of a negative impact on daily life. This can lead to improved mood, reduced stress, and better overall well-being.
   - <u>Empowerment</u>: Successfully managing exposure to previously triggering sounds can empower individuals, giving them a sense of control over their environment and their reactions.

Psychological Benefits

1. ***Building Resilience***
   - *Confidence Growth*: Each successful exposure session builds resilience and confidence, reinforcing the belief that one can handle challenging sounds.
   - *Decreased Avoidance*: As tolerance improves, individuals may find themselves less likely to avoid social situations or environments where loud sounds are present, leading to a fuller, more engaged life.

2. ***Stress Reduction***
   - *Relaxation Techniques*: Incorporating relaxation techniques during breaks and before sessions can further aid in reducing stress and anxiety, creating a holistic approach to managing sound sensitivity.
   - *Mindfulness Practices*: Mindfulness and meditation practices can complement sound sensitivity training by helping individuals remain calm and centered, further reducing the impact of triggering sounds.

Practical Application

1. ***Daily Integration***
   - *Routine Practice*: Regularly practicing exposure exercises can make dealing with real-world

noise less daunting. Integrating these exercises into daily routines ensures continuous progress.
- *Environmental Control*: Starting in a controlled environment allows for adjustments based on immediate feedback, fine-tuning the approach for optimal comfort and effectiveness.

2. **Support Systems**
   - *Professional Guidance*: Working with a therapist who specializes in misophonia or sound sensitivity can provide personalized strategies and support, enhancing the effectiveness of the training.
   - *Community Support*: Joining support groups or online forums can offer additional motivation and shared experiences, reinforcing the commitment to the training process.

By understanding and applying these principles, sound sensitivity training can be a powerful tool in managing and overcoming noise anxiety. The gradual and controlled exposure, combined with changes in perception and the integration of relaxation techniques, offers a comprehensive approach to improving the quality of life for those with sound sensitivity.

Talk to Friends and Family

Talk to your family and friends. Misophonia can be hard to deal with, but you don't have to go through it alone.

Talk to your family and friends about your condition and let them know what they can do to help you. For example, you might ask them to be more aware of the sounds they make or to avoid making certain sounds around you.

The reason why talking to friends and family helps is that they will be more understanding and accommodating of your condition. If they know that a certain sound bothers you, they will be more likely to avoid making that noise.

The science of talking to friends and family is a topic that has been studied by researchers for many years. The act of talking to someone you know and care about can have a positive impact on your mood and overall well-being. In fact, research has shown that social support can help reduce stress, improve mental and physical health, and even increase lifespan.

There are several reasons why talking to friends and family can be beneficial. First, it allows you to share your thoughts and feelings with someone who cares about you. This can help reduce stress by providing an outlet for your emotions. Additionally, talking openly with others can help build trust and intimacy, which are important ingredients for healthy relationships. Finally, social support can provide a sense of belongingness and connectedness, which can boost self-esteem and overall satisfaction with life.

Another benefit of talking to your friends and family is that it can help to reduce the stigma surrounding misophonia. When you talk about your condition, it helps to normalize it and makes it more acceptable.

If you're not comfortable talking to your friends and family about your condition, there are other ways to get support. There are online forums and support groups for people with misophonia. These can be a great way to connect with others who understand what you're going through. Some examples of online forums include:

1. The Misophonia Association
2. Reddit's /r/misophonia
3. The International Misophonia Research Network

While online forums can be a great way to connect with others, it's important to remember that not everyone will have the same experience as you. Take what you read with a grain of salt and don't be afraid to reach out to a professional if you need help.

Conclusion

Thank you for taking the time to read our guide on misophonia. By now, you should have a clearer understanding of what misophonia is, how it affects daily life, and some strategies you can use to manage it effectively.

Living with misophonia can be tough, but remember, you're not alone. Many people deal with this condition and have found ways to cope successfully. The key is to recognize your triggers early and take proactive steps to lessen their impact. You've already made great progress by learning about misophonia, and that's a significant step forward.

One important insight to keep in mind is the value of self-awareness and self-care. Knowing what sounds trigger your misophonia allows you to create environments that help reduce stress. Simple actions like using noise-canceling headphones, practicing relaxation techniques, or joining supportive communities can make a big difference in your daily life.

It's also crucial to communicate your needs to those around you. Friends, family members, and colleagues might not know much about misophonia, but once they understand your situation, they are likely to be more supportive. Don't be afraid to explain your condition and suggest ways they can help, like reducing certain noises or being mindful of their actions.

If you find it hard to manage misophonia on your own, seeking professional help can be very beneficial. Therapists and counselors specializing in sensory processing disorders can offer personalized strategies and emotional support. Cognitive-behavioral therapy (CBT) has shown promise in helping individuals change their responses to triggering sounds.

Staying connected with others who have similar experiences can also provide comfort and practical advice. Online forums, support groups, and social media communities dedicated to misophonia can be valuable resources. Sharing your journey and hearing others' stories can remind you that overcoming the challenges of misophonia is possible.

As you continue your journey, be patient with yourself. Progress might be slow, but every small step counts. Celebrate your victories, no matter how minor they seem, and remember that it's okay to seek help when needed.

In conclusion, managing misophonia involves finding a balance between avoidance, confrontation, and acceptance. You have the power to shape your environment and your responses in ways that promote well-being. By adopting effective coping mechanisms and maintaining open communication, you can lead a fulfilling and less stressful life.

Once again, thank you for reading this guide. Your commitment to understanding and managing misophonia shows your strength and determination. Keep pushing forward, stay informed, and most importantly, be kind to yourself.

Sample Worksheets

Trigger Sound List	Sensitivity Rate	Frequency Exercise	Notes

FAQs

What is misophonia?

Misophonia is a condition where certain sounds trigger strong emotional reactions such as anger, anxiety, or disgust. Common triggers include sounds like chewing, tapping, or breathing. These reactions can disrupt daily life and cause significant distress.

What are the common symptoms of misophonia?

People with misophonia often experience intense emotional responses to specific sounds. Symptoms may include irritability, anger, anxiety, discomfort, and the urge to escape the triggering sound. Physical reactions like sweating or an increased heart rate can also occur.

How is misophonia diagnosed?

There is no official medical test for diagnosing misophonia. Diagnosis typically involves a thorough evaluation by a healthcare professional who will consider your symptoms, and their impact on your life, and rule out other possible conditions. Describing your triggers and reactions in detail can help in the assessment process.

What strategies can help manage misophonia?

Effective strategies for managing misophonia include using noise-canceling headphones, creating a quiet environment, practicing relaxation techniques, and seeking support from friends, family, or support groups. Cognitive-behavioral therapy (CBT) has also been shown to help some individuals reframe their responses to triggering sounds.

Can misophonia be treated?

While there is no cure for misophonia, various treatments and coping strategies can help manage the condition. Therapies like CBT, sound therapy, and counseling can provide significant relief. It's important to work with a healthcare professional to find the best approach for your situation.

How can I explain misophonia to others?

When explaining misophonia, it's helpful to describe it as a heightened sensitivity to specific sounds that trigger strong emotional reactions. You can share examples of your triggers and explain how they affect you. Encourage understanding and suggest ways others can help, such as reducing certain noises or being mindful of their actions.

Are there any support groups for people with misophonia?

Yes, there are several online forums, social media groups, and local support groups dedicated to misophonia. These communities can provide valuable advice, share personal experiences, and offer emotional support. Connecting with others who understand what you're going through can be very comforting and helpful.

References and Helpful Links

Eijsker, N., Schröder, A., Smit, D. J., Van Wingen, G., & Denys, D. (2021). Structural and functional brain abnormalities in misophonia. European Neuropsychopharmacology, 52, 62–71. https://doi.org/10.1016/j.euroneuro.2021.05.013

Arthur, A. (n.d.). Misophonia: Scientists discover the brain connection responsible for "supersensitivity" to noise. BBC Science Focus Magazine. https://www.sciencefocus.com/news/misophonia-scientists-discover-the-brain-connection-responsible-for-supersensitivity-to-noise

Evans, J. R. (2023, March 14). Understanding misophonia: when everyday sounds cause distress. Healthline. https://www.healthline.com/health/misophonia

Cartreine, J., PhD. (2019, June 24). Misophonia: When sounds really do make you "crazy." Harvard Health. https://www.health.harvard.edu/blog/misophonia-sounds-really-make-crazy-2017042111534

Schröder, A., Van Wingen, G., Eijsker, N., Giorgi, R. S., Vulink, N. C., Turbyne, C., & Denys, D. (2019). Misophonia is associated with altered brain activity in the auditory cortex and salience network. Scientific Reports, 9(1). https://doi.org/10.1038/s41598-019-44084-8

Cuncic, A., MA. (2023, July 25). Overview of misophonia treatment. Verywell Mind. https://www.verywellmind.com/misophonia-treatment-4845902#:~:text=Several%20types%20of%20behavioral%20treatment,strategies%20to%20manage%20negative%20reactions.

Hübscher, C. R., & Hübscher, C. R. (2023, September 11). Why do I hate certain noises? (Misophonia CBT therapy). GroundWork Counseling. https://www.groundworkcounseling.com/anxiety/why-do-i-hate-certain-noises-misophonia/

www.ingramcontent.com/pod-product-compliance
Lightning Source LLC
LaVergne TN
LVHW012036060526
838201LV00061B/4627